POTPIE DIET

SAVE TIME
SAVE MONEY
LOSE WEIGHT

BARB DOYON

To readers:

This book contains opinions and ideas of the author. It is intended to provide helpful information on the subject matter. It is sold with the understanding that the author is not rendering medical or health advice and the reader should always consult a physician before beginning any diet plan. The author specifically disclaim all responsibility for any liability, loss, or risk, personal or otherwise, which is incurred as a consequence, directly or indirectly, of the use and application of any of the contents of this book.

Front & Back Cover Photography Licensed by Pond5.com
Interior Design by Soumi Goswami

BARB DOYON is an award-winning documentary film writer, author, producer & story analyst who resides in Los Angeles, California. After years of struggling with weight, she adapted her great grandmother's potpie recipes into do-it-yourself, pre-packaged, low-fat, low-calorie meal plans that allowed her to enjoy comfort foods and resulted in a 57-pound weight loss in 8 months.

CONTENTS

CHAPTER 1

BACK TO BASICS

BEEN THERE, DONE THAT

How many diets have you failed? If you're reading this book, the answer is obvious, all of them. And that's a lot of diets. There are the pre-packaged food diets, the pill diets, the low-carb diets, the low-calorie diets, the no-fat diets, the low-fat diets, the vegan diets, the shake diets and so on. Like you, I've tried them all. Frankly, I appreciate the pre-packaged diet plans because they save me the most time and I don't have to count, weigh, measure or add up points. But one downside is the cost. And, while I like most of the food, one popular brand has dinners that I find nasty and another brand has breakfasts that taste like paste. If I don't like a meal, I'm stuck with it. And what happens after I've lost weight and have to deal with real-world foods? As for the other diets, I find it hard to believe that if I eat carbs I'll get fat. If this were the case, then how to people lose weight-eating Subway sandwiches several times a day?

The diet world is riddled with contradictory information of what works and what doesn't work. The reality is that most diets hold the promise of some weight loss. I've personally lost an average of ten pounds on each of the many diets I've tried, only to gain back twelve pounds.

Then, one day, I went back home for a visit. While I currently reside in Los Angeles, California, I grew up in backwoods of Pennsylvania. While visiting an elderly aunt, she served white bread sandwiches laden with mayo and cucumbers, potato chips and black coffee. I'm from L.A., we don't eat this stuff, but I wouldn't dream of insulting an elder, so I ate white bread and mayo for the first time in years and it's probably only the third cup of coffee I've ever drank. I'm a tea drinker.

It was then that something occurred to me. My aunt is 87 years old and she's bouncing around her kitchen serving lunch with more energy than I have most of the day! I started to think about all the relatives from the old country: the grandparents, great grandparents, the aunts and uncles. They all lived to be in their 80's and 90's and none of them were fat. In fact, I was the plumpest one at the table. How'd that happen? What was I missing? More importantly, what was I doing wrong?

Well, in all fairness, the elders didn't live the sedentary lifestyle we do today. They manned the farms, tended the gardens, hiked the woods for game to put meat on the table, and if they needed a gallon of milk they'd walk the mile to the nearest store to get it. Today, we'd get in the car and drive to the store for milk, even if the store's only a block away. Let's face it, we live in our cars, in front of our TV sets, behind a desk tucked into a cubicle, and have iPhones glued to our ears like permanent fixtures. We're the poster generation for the sedentary lifestyle and it's huge part of the reason we're overweight.

While a sedentary lifestyle certainly plays a big role in obesity, the fact is that the elders ate bacon every day and used the bacon grease to flavor foods like potatoes, rice, soups, etc. They ate white bread with every meal: homemade rolls, biscuits, pancakes, sandwiches, cakes, and pies. And yet they were rarely overweight.

But wait a minute. I'm forgetting something. Most of the foods they consumed came from their own gardens or from wild sources in the forest, like blackberries, raspberries and walnuts. They grew everything garden fresh like rhubarb, pumpkins, potatoes, cucumbers, beets, corn, carrots, sunflowers, wheat, watermelons, herbs, radishes, peas, etc. They also had land filled with fruit trees: cherry, peach, apple, lemons, lime and fig.

I could only conclude that the elders' physically healthy lifestyle and a combination of good/bad foods were the contributing factors to slimness and longevity. By good/bad foods I mean the garden fresh goodness mixed with what we'd consider the bad stuff, the breads, the fats, the red meats, etc. Let's face it, they had a healthy balance that today's society struggles to recreate with places that provide garden fresh produce, like organic markets and places that provide physical fitness, like gyms.

I realize there's no going back to the good old days, but I began to think that there might be a way to tap into the wisdom of the elders and adapt it to fit today's busy lifestyle and it starts with my great grandmother's potpie recipe.

OLD SCHOOL WAYS

Long before Jenny Craig, Nutrisystem or any other pre-packaged food systems came along, my great grandmother was pre-packaging foods the old school way. When it came to food, she was a master at saving time and money. And food never went to waste in her house. I'd help her roll out different types of dough like bread dough, pizza dough, pie dough, etc., and we'd bake up all kinds of wonderful, homemade treats. But she didn't stop there. She'd take the baked goods and freeze them!

ELDERS USED TO PRE-MAKE FOOD

The one I remember with most fondness were her potpies. She made chicken potpies; beef potpies, vegetable potpies, pork potpies, scrambled egg potpies, and many other varieties that covered breakfast, lunch and dinner. She'd cut up produce from the garden during the week and chopped meats into bite-sized pieces in the evenings. Then on the weekend and put all the ingredients into potpies, mixed with soups, cheeses, vegetables, herbs, and other ingredients. She'd make dozens at a time, freeze them and for the next few weeks, or even months during the wintertime, we'd eat the hearty potpies up to three times a day. I loved the scrambled egg, bacon and cheese potpies for breakfast, the meatloaf potpies for dinner the fruit-filled potpie-style cobblers for dessert. All we had to do was reheat the potpies in the microwave or oven and eat them. It was good, old-fashioned comfort foods that left you feeling satisfied. Best of all, we saved time and money by preparing the pies ahead and by making them homemade.

But can this old school way be adapted to today's lifestyle? Let's face it; grandma's recipes were laden with enough fat to send the average 40-year-old man to the emergency room in cardiac arrest after a single day of residing in potpie heaven. And with today's busy lifestyles, do we really have time to prep our own food? Let's find out.

HOW TO SAVE TIME & MONEY

It goes without saying that if you make food at home, as opposed to eating out, that you save money. The amount can be into the hundreds or even more depending on how often you eat out. And while restaurants provide nutritional information that includes calorie and fat counts, the only way to really know what's in something is if you make it.

Don't worry; you don't have to know how to cook! This book is going to show you a fast, simple and easy way to incorporate the Potpie Diet into your busy lifestyle.

What about time? Who has time to make potpies? This is a valid question. Most of us are struggling to find more time in our lives. If you add up the time spent making breakfast, lunch and dinner seven days a week, how much time does that add up to? Let's economize and say you spend an hour a day between breakfast, lunch and dinner. That's roughly seven hours a week or almost the same time you spend at one day at your job. Yikes!

What if you could reduce that time to one hour a week? You'd have six extra hours a week to play, read, study, relax, sleep, take a hike, visit friends & family, go on a picnic, or enjoy the great outdoors.

Is one hour a week really realistic? Yes and this book will show you how to make it happen.

FAT FACTOR

What about the fact that potpies are laden with high calories, fat and other things we consider bad by today's standards? This book is going to show you how to make healthy, tasty potpies that will save you time, money and assist you with weight loss by reducing portion size and fat intake. We're literally going to modernize grandma's potpies. And best of all, you'll be creating a comfort food that appeals to your own pallet rather than hoping that the pre-packaged meal you purchased doesn't offend your taste buds. Or purchasing store bought potpies that might have a lower calorie count (although most break the diet bank) and are filled with fatty fats.

CHAPTER 2

SETTING GOALS

HOW MUCH DO YOU REALLY NEED TO LOSE?

Before starting any diet and exercise plan, you should consult with a physician. The first thing you need to do is figure out exactly how much you need to lose. Don't guess. You're probably wrong. Let's keep this simple. Start by figuring out your Body Mass Index (BMI), then your Basal Metabolic Rate (BMR), which will help you determine your daily calorie intake. It's important to know your daily-allotted calorie intake so you don't go over and end up gaining weight while you're trying to lose it. This shouldn't be an issue with the Potpie Diet because it'll always leaving you feeling satisfied.

The easiest way to figure out this information is to go on-line. There are plenty of BMI and BMR calculators that will do the math for you. If you'd rather do it by hand or with a calculator, here are the steps:

BODY MASS INDEX (BMI) CALCULATOR

To calculate your Body Mass Index (BMI), do the following:

1. Weigh yourself, preferably with a reliable, digital scale.
2. Multiply your weight by 703.
3. Divide the answer by your height in inches.
4. Divide that answer again by your height in inches.

For example, a 150-pound person who is 5'5" tall would do the calculations as follows:

150 x 703 = 105,450

105,450/65 (height in inches) = 1622.30

1622.30/65 = 24.95 BMI

BASAL METABOLIC RATE (BMR) CALCULATOR

To calculate your Basal Metabolic Rate (BMR), do the following:

1. For Women: Multiply your weight by 4.35, your height in inches by 4.7 and your age by 4.7. For a 40-year-old woman at 5'6" and 150 lbs., you would have the following (150 x 4.35 = 652.5), (66 x 4.7 = 310.2), (40 x 4.7 = 188). Add 655 to the height and weight and subtract your age: 655 + 310.2 – 188 = a BMR of 1,430 (1,429.7).

2. For Men: Multiple your weight by 6.23, your height, in inches, by 12.7, and your age by 6.8. For a 40-year-old man at 5'6" and 150 lbs., you would have the following: (150 x 6.23 = 934.5), (66 x 12.7= 838.2), (40 x 6.8 = 272). Add 66 to the height and weight and subtract your age: 66 + 934.5 + 838.2 – 272 = a BMR of 1,567 (1,566.7).

DAILY CALORIE INTAKE CALCUATOR

To calculate your daily calorie intake, do the following:

1. Determine your activity level:

   Sedentary/Multiply BMR by 1.2

   Lightly Active/Multiply BMR by 1.375

   Moderately Active/Multiply BMR by 1.55

   Very Active/Multiple BMR by 1.725

   Extra Active/Multiply BMR by 1.9

2. For example, a moderately active man would use the following equation: 1,567 x 1.55 = a maximum of 2,429 calories a day.

HOW LONG WILL IT TAKE?

This can be the most painful part because most of you want to lose weight yesterday. You want it fast; 5 or more pounds a week and you usually start out with a bang, averaging 5 or more pounds in the first week, most of which is water loss, not fat. The problem with fast weight loss is fast weight gain. Your body thinks it's starving and the moment you stop dieting the fat piles back on with a few extra pounds just in case you're dumb enough to try that again. Your body has this built-in survival mechanism. Fight it and you'll lose.

Instead, get realistic. Is losing 1 to 2 pounds a week really that bad? I'm no fan of numbers, but let's do the math. At 2 pounds a week that's 8 pounds per month. Time flies and before you know it three months have gone by and wow, now you're at 24 pounds of weight loss! When is the last time you lost a solid 24 pounds? And, the best part is, you're still losing!

It's like the elders always said, SLOW AND STEADY WINS THE RACE!

ELIMINATE THE JUNK FOOD

The easiest ways to sabotage your efforts is to have the bad stuff nearby. By nearby, I mean in your house within arms reach. Do you really want to lose 15 pounds, then get a salt craving and end up eating an entire bag of potato chips? Or a sugar craving and end up eating a half-a-box of cookies?

While I personally believe that eating the hearty, comfort foods in the Potpie Diet will help you maintain a balance to prevent cravings, we're all different and cravings can and do happen. Women have monthly hormonal changes that can cause them to raid a refrigerator and men might be stressed and finish off a plate of nachos dripping with cheese sauce and greasy ground beef.

The best way to assure you can meet these challenging times is to eliminate the junk food.

GET IT OUT OF YOUR HOUSE

GET IT OUT OF YOUR LIFE

GET IT OUT OF YOUR SIGHT

This way it won't end up in your mouth! I already know what you're going to say, 'I keep it in the house because the kids like it.' I bet if I surveyed the kids, they'd tell me that you're the one who eats most of it! Come on! It's time to really do this. If you want fast food that comforts whatever is making you binge in the first place, then turn to the healthy options first and use the potpies to help you stay satisfied so you won't feel like diving into the next box of donuts you walk by.

By the way, kids need to eat healthier too. Do you want them eating candy bars or apples? If eating healthy is so important to you, then why isn't it important for your kids? It should be. Eliminate the junk food and replace it with fresh, healthy alternatives.

I realize there are compulsive eaters who eat due to stress, boredom, out of anxiety or for other reasons, but isn't it time to deal with these issues head on instead of with food? Get out the metaphorical boxing gloves and knock out whatever is causing the stress. Fight boredom with hobbies and activities you love to do. You know the ones you keep complaining you never have enough time to do. Eliminate anxiety with exercise not food – see Chapter 5 and Get Moving!

CHAPTER 3

GET MOVING!

EXERCISE SHOULD BE A 4-LETTER WORD

You hate to exercise. Join the club! It's hard. It's time consuming. It hurts. The excuses not to exercise are boundless; you don't have time in the morning because you have to get the kids off to school, walk the dog, make lunches, make breakfast, shower and get ready for work. During the day, you're at work. When you finally arrive home in the evening, after a long day, fighting rush hour traffic, you're dead tired and you still have to make dinner and get ready for tomorrow. There's simply no time to exercise. Oh wait, you'll go on a nice walk on the weekend.

I'm not going to argue with you. You're right. Life is time consuming. We're lucky to have enough hours to sleep let alone spend 30-minutes, several times a week exercising. And I don't want you to think of exercise as a chore you have to do if you want to lose weight. Frankly, you can lose weight just by cutting out calories and fat, but is weight loss all you really want? Don't you want to look and feel great? Well, guess what, that's where the exercise part comes in.

DO YOU JUST WANT TO LOSE WEIGHT?
OR DO YOU WANT TO LOOK & FEEL GREAT TOO?

Obviously, exercise can help you lose weight at a faster pace and keep it off. But it can also help you sculpt your body into the finely tuned image you want to see when you look in the mirror. And most importantly, the health benefits of exercise are enormous from lowering blood pressure, blood sugar, high cholesterol, reducing stress, releasing endorphins that helps you feel better, relieving anxiety and boredom, etc.

But let's be realistic, most of you already know this and you still haven't budged off the couch. So I say – stay on the couch! What? Let me rephrase by saying, start on the couch. That is, start exercising on the couch.

COUCH POTATO'S EXERCISE PLAN

So, you're a confessed couch potato who won't give up the remote control easily. To hell with exercise, but okay, you want to lose weight, look great and feel better, so you'll give this Couch Potato Exercise Plan a try. Great!

First, let's start with the basics, stretching. It's pretty easy to stretch your arms and legs while sitting on the couch. Start there. Do a few reps, then stretch your neck and back a few times. That wasn't so hard, was it?

Let's take this to the next level. Don't worry; you can stay on the couch – for now. Since we've already discussed a lot of old school things, I personally like Suzanne Somers Thigh Master and did you know she also has a Butt Master? You can get a full body workout with these two gems. Maybe this isn't your thing. Okay, then try weights. You can buy 2-5 pound hand weight or strap-on, Velcro weights at any Wal-Mart or Target. Do arm and leg exercises on the couch with your Suzanne Somers Toning System and/or the weights, and then you can proudly say you've mastered the art of Couch Potato Exercising.

But something else is going to happen along the way. You're going to start to like the way you look and feel. You're going to want more.

BUILD UP TO BODY BUILDING

Stick with the toning and weights on the couch, but take it up a notch. Don't worry; you don't have to leave the living room, yet. Next step is to get off the couch and march in place.

That's right, I said MARCH, not walk, not run, but march. After months of trying to lose weight, I watched my police sergeant neighbor lose 20 pounds in a month by doing nothing but marching in place with a baton. No, it wasn't a magic baton. He just marched in place in his back yard and you know what, it works because it gets the arms and legs moving, while raising the heart rate and burning calories. Best of all, you don't have to miss a single episode of your favorite TV show.

But you feel silly marching in place in front of your wife, your husband, your kids, your dog or your cat. Well, I have a cat and a dog and I can guarantee you they don't care. As for the family, you work hard, pay the bills and you deserve to look and feel your best. If they don't like it, tell them to find another room in the house to hang out in or they can join you!

MARCH IN PLACE

When you start seeing the results of the Potpie Diet, the toning, weights and marching in place, you're going to want more. That's the great thing about exercise, it's like a drug that works; once you see the results you want more of the cure until you're completely well again! Now it's time to move up to bodybuilding. Aerobics are great, but they're really more for cardiovascular. I once overheard a trainer say that he never saw anyone lose weight using a treadmill. I don't know if this is entirely accurate because I believe any form of body movement for 30-minutes or more consistently is good for you, but I do know from personal experience that the fastest, easiest way to sculpt a new you is with bodybuilding.

SCULPT A NEW YOU

Yes, I'm talking about weight training. Not that kind that makes you big, like the Incredible Hulk. Weight training can help you trim down your waist while widening your shoulders to give you an ultra-slim appearance. Or slim down your thighs while building muscles in your arms. With weights, your body's like a piece of clay that can be molded into a desired shape.

Do not try this yourself. Have a trainer help you. I know what you're thinking. I can't afford a gym, let alone a trainer. Well, the gym will run you around $30 a month. If you cut out the junk food, you should be able to swing $30 a month. However, I realize the cost of the trainer might be out of your range, so here's what you do. Ask the gym's manager (or a trainer) for a demonstration on how to use the weight training equipment. Most gyms will do this for free. If not, then splurge on a 30-minute to 1-hour session. Learning how to properly use weights is the key to learning to sculpt your body.

Before you get trained in weights, really hone in on what you want to know. For example, because I write so much my upper back and neck gets tense. I asked the trainer, in a free, gym-provided demonstration, which equipment to use to strengthen my back and neck muscles to help eliminate future problems. He was happy to show me. Think beyond the skinny thighs and really target what you need to look and feel your best. Of course, be sure to have the trainer show you how to get skinny thighs too, then your neck/back will feel great and you'll look great.

MOVE YOUR BODY
30-MINUTES CONSISTENTLY
3-TIMES A WEEK

Important Note: The key to losing weight is to get your body moving for 30 consistent minutes at least 3 times a week, but I think you'll find that once you start looking and feeling better that the 30 minutes turns into an hour and 3 times a week turns into 5, 6, 7.

WATER, WATER, WATER

Oprah Winfrey says she hates drinking water, so she drinks her entire daily dose each morning to get it out of the way. Okay, if that works for you then fine. But getting in those 8 glasses a day is imperative to weight loss and proper bodily functions. But like you and Oprah, I don't like drinking water either. I'm a tea connoisseur and I admit I like an occasional soda pop.

The best way I've found to get in the necessary water intake daily is to make it taste better. Most of you use lemon or limes, but this is outdated and doesn't match the comfort level we're seeking as part of the Potpie Diet. Instead, try what I call the Frozen Fruit approach.

I cut up oranges, pineapple, kiwis, strawberries, grapes and other favorite, juicy fruits, tuck them into a large freeze bag and freeze them. Then when it's time for a glass of water, I add pieces of the frozen fruit instead of ice. As the fruit thaws, it gives the water a mellow fruit flavor and when I'm done drinking, I eat the fruit. Yummy!

USE FROZEN FRUIT
IN PLACE OF ICE CUBES
FOR A REFRESHING, TASTY
ALTERNATIVE TO DRINKING WATER

This is also a great treat in the summer. Try frozen red and white grapes. They're a cool treat on a hot summer's day.

STRESS RELIEF

There are too many techniques for stress relief to cover in a dozen books, so let's try a different approach and focus on stress relief during your most stressful, daily moments. For many, it's driving to work in bumper-to-bumper, rush hour traffic. There are audio book selections, music or even listening to a seminar (the one you missed because you were too busy working and had to buy the download).

Household stress is tough to get away from. There are the screaming kids, the grumpy spouse or the annoying, nosy neighbor. Expand the marching in place to the outdoors. Get away from it all for 30-minutes. If your family finds excuses to sabotage your efforts by telling you that you can't go for a walk when the trash needs taken out or the lawn mowed or the kitchen sink fixed, then adopt a dog. Then you can tell your family that you have no choice. You have to take a walk because Fido has to go to the bathroom! By the way, pets can be great stress relief. They're loyal, loving and no matter how long you're gone for work they'll still be they're waiting when you get home.

EXERCISE
LISTEN TO MUSIC

LISTEN TO AUDIO BOOKS
READ A BOOK
ADOPT A PET
GO FOR A WALK

Warning: Don't ignore stress relief. Stress is a contributing factor to weight gain among many other health issues. Life is short. Try to avoid, eliminate or reduce stress from your life as much as possible

CHAPTER 4

POTPIE DIET

GETTING STARTED

Getting started on The Potpie Diet is fast and easy. By now, you should have cleared out the junk food from the cupboards. Now it's time to focus on the freezer. Start by clearing the freezer of junk foods like ice cream, frozen pies, TV dinners and anything else that you know is a deal breaker on your quest to looking and feeling great. You're doing this to eliminate temptation and to make room for The Potpie Diet.

Next, you'll need potpie containers. This part can be tricky. Pay close attention to portion size. I'd recommend going with…

Pantry Elements Silicone Baking Cups (3.5 inch size)
Quantity: 12 available at Amazon.com

Or try this alternative:

Casabella 4-inch Large Baking Cup. Set of 6 assorted colors.
Dimensions: 4-inch, 1.75-inch x 4-inches.

These are the preferred containers because they're safe for baking, microwave, freezer and dishwasher. There are toss-out-after-use, foil options, like Eco-Foil's Mini Loaf Pans (size 5in. x 3in x 1in), but you can't heat up the potpies in the microwave and you'll have to transfer the potpie to another container first. Since the goal is to save time, it's recommended you go with a versatile container that works in the freezer, oven, microwave and dishwasher. And it's easy to take with you for lunches at work or for family outings. Plus, you'll be able to reuse the Pantry Elements Silicone Baking Cups, which will save money.

The key is to keep the portion size of the container under 5inches at the widest point.

Also, stock up on paper cupcake liners. They're perfect for making mini potpies and cobblers.

GROCERY LIST

Make the same list you always make for the grocery store, but let's take a good, hard look at it. The typical list has bread, eggs, milk, meat, vegetables, rice, pasta, mashed potatoes, frozen pizzas, TV dinners, donuts and other assorted diet breakers.

First, identify the comfort foods on your list. It's okay to admit you can't live without pizza. The Potpie Diet has a Pizza For Breakfast recipe! It's okay to admit you'd rather have a hamburger and fries for lunch than a salad. The Potpie Diet has a hamburger and fries recipe! It's okay to admit you'd rather have a Shepherd's Potpie for dinner than fish. The Potpie Diet has a recipe for Shepherd's Potpie! If you want the fish, the Potpie Diet has a Tuna Potpie recipe. Get the picture? On this diet you don't have to give up the foods you love, but you will need to learn to modify them in a way that provides a lower calorie count and smaller portion size to fit your daily caloric intake.

Does this mean you can diet without salads, vegetables, fruits, etc.? NO! It means you're going to layer your comfort foods with the other foods to ease the burden of dieting. And to prevent you from quitting like you've done on so many other diets in the past.

LEAN & LOW-FAT = LESS CALORIES

The trick to keeping your comfort foods is to make different choices of the same foods you love. For example, if you love everything smothered in cheese, then instead of selecting the regular cheese, select a low-fat (2% milk fat) cheese. The lower calorie and fat count will allow you to continue to enjoy cheese, in moderation, without packing on the pounds.

Do the same for other foods you love. Instead of fried chicken, pick the rotisserie chicken, flame-broiled or baked. Instead of fatty ground, select 80% or higher lean beef or go with ground turkey. Never drink whole milk again. Go with the 2% variety. If you love mashed potatoes, make them with chicken broth instead of butter. By the way, butter is a major deal breaker and while it can be used in extreme moderation, its fat content can sink any diet ship. If you find you simply can't live without the comfort of butter, then try brands like I Can't Believe It's Not Butter.

Fresh vegetables are preferred over frozen, but they can take up prep time. I'd recommend Green Giant's Steamers Healthy Weight selections. They're pre-packaged with low-fat and low-calorie counts. Many are made with light butter sauces and creamy dressings, which are perfect comfort foods to add to The Potpie Diet.

Try to add more fish to your diet. Forget anything that has breading. I prefer pre-cooked selections like tilapia, salmon and shrimp. For tuna, always choose 'packed in water' over 'packed in oil' to significantly reduce the fat and calorie count.

Be careful not to drink calories. Extra calories that can sabotage a diet can be hidden in soda pop, teas, coffees, sports drinks, juices, etc. For now, I'd recommend reducing these beverages to 1-2 per day and be sure to add in the calories consumed to your overall diet plan.

If you're not used to doing this, plan an extra 30-minutes in the store. Give yourself enough time to really look at the labels and to really understand what you're buying and how it'll affect your overall diet plan.

What if you have been doing this, but still haven't lost weight? Then, my best guess is that you have an issue with portion size and/or going over your daily caloric intake, either of which can add pounds.

ITEMS TO ADD TO THE GROCERY LIST

For The Potpie Diet, you'll need to add a mandatory item to your list, the potpie crust. What would a potpie be without a warm, delicious crust? But who has time to roll out a crust? Nobody and your goal is to save time, not to waste it covered in flour and beating a rolling pin against a tabletop.

Head straight to the freeze section of the grocery store and find the Pillsbury dough section. You can certainly make a different selection, but the calorie count on Pillsbury's freezer dough fits The Potpie Diet to perfection. Here are the choices:

Pillsbury, refrigerated Crescent Rolls – Qty. 8

Pillsbury, refrigerated Pie Crust – 1 box

Pillsbury, refrigerated Pizza Crust – 1 box

(Note: Pillsbury also offers Gluten free dough)

You can buy the biscuits too, but be careful because they have the highest calorie count and will require you to cut back on the other selections when you put your pie together.

FOR BISCUIT-STYLE CRUST
USE BETTY CROCKER BISCUIT MIX

If you prefer a biscuit crust, then go with Betty Crocker's Biscuit Mix. Buy a few packages so you'll have enough for a few weeks.

Secondly, the Pie Crust will require you to roll it out. Same goes with the Pizza Crust, so the best choice and it's the lowest calorie count is the Pillsbury, refrigerated Crescent Rolls – Quantity 8. They're pre-cut, ready to go and each package has 8. You'll learn why this is important in a minute.

I realize most of you will grow tired of the potpies crust pretty fast, probably after 1-2 weeks, so get creative with the crust. Use properly portioned Corn Flakes (see box for portion sizes, calorie count), low-fat cheese, chopped nuts, fruits, and other low-fat, low-calorie options. Be creative. But stay away from fatty, high calorie crusts that can sabotage your efforts, like graham crusts and high-fat cheeses.

This diet is also going to offer options to the potpies that are fast, easy and fit the main philosophy of the diet; fast, easy, on-the-go comfort foods that save time, money and help you lose weight.

Next, let's focus on the creamy insides of the potpies! This is where most diets would fail, but like you've already been taught, you'll be substituting the high-fat, high-calorie, diet busters for sensible options that will allow you to enjoy your favorite, comfort foods.

Add to your grocery list Campbell's Soup Selections. You can choose from your favorites: Cream of Chicken, Cream of Mushroom, Cream of Mushroom with Roasted Garlic or Cream of Celery. There are 98% fat free options, but this isn't really necessary because the regular Cream of Mushroom soup is only 60 calories for a ½ cup portion, which is what you'll need per potpie serving. Perfect!

Extra soup note: I don't add water to the soup. This keeps the potpies thick, creamy and delicious.

DO NOT ADD WATER TO THE SOUPS
THIS MAKES THE POTPIE CREAMY

You should be able to get at least 2 portions out of each can and you'll be making food for the week, so purchase 4 cans of your favorites.

PORTION SIZE

Most of you don't have time to count, weigh and measure foods. The Potpie Diet does have some measuring involved, but it's mostly in the prep phase. Once your potpies are prepped, all you have to do is heat and eat. No measuring, weighing, counting or worrying and most importantly, no starving because you'll be eating the comfort foods you craved on other diets.

The first trick to this diet was choosing lean & low-fat foods that equal lower calories. The second trick is portion size. By sticking to the recommend potpie container (see section under Chapter 4: Getting Started), you'll be able to keep portions under control. This isn't a new trick. The pre-packaged diet giants with their celebrity endorsements have been doing it for years. And while they offer a fast, easy solution, it'll cost you and if you select a meal you don't like you're stuck with it. Frankly, my biggest concern with these plans is what happens after you lose weight and start eating real-world food again?

With The Potpie Diet, you're pre-packaging comfort foods you selected that you love. You're keeping costs down by doing it yourself (1 hour a week) and when you lose weight you'll never have to worry about having to deal with real-world foods because you're already eating real-world, comfort foods EVERY DAY!

QUANTITY SAVES TIME & MONEY

You've made your regular grocery list. You've modified it with low-fat, low calories selections of your favorite, comfort foods and purchased the pre-made crust of your choice. You've purchased potpie containers to assure the proper portion size. The next phase of the diet is the prep.

YOU ONLY NEED ONE HOUR A WEEK!

For most of you, that's a weekend day, either Saturday or Sunday. Since the first thing I do each day is eat breakfast, I start by preparing the breakfast selections that I'll be freezing for the Potpie Diet. I cook seven portions of egg whites (or egg beaters) and seven turkey sausages and set these aside with a small bowl of low-fat cheese. I use one Pillsbury, refrigerated Crescent roll package (8 total rolls). Remove the rolls and tear apart along the seams. Fill each with one with equal portions of egg, one turkey sausage and a pinch of cheese. Bake in over according to the temperature and time on the Crescent Roll package. Remove, cool, wrap and freeze. You now have breakfast for 7 days, prepped, portioned and ready to eat. The calorie count is 350. It's okay to make 8. Use the extra for next week or give it to the kids or feed the family pet a breakfast snack.

YOU CAN FIND ALL THE RECIPES FOR
BREAKFAST, LUNCH & DINNER
ALONG WITH MEAL PLANS
IN THE CHAPTERS UNDER MEAL PLANS & RECIPES

Next, I prep lunch and dinner at the same time. Decide on what meats and vegetables you'd like in your potpies. Maybe you'd like a chicken potpie for lunch and a Shepherd's potpie for dinner. When you were at the store, you bought a rotisserie chicken and lean ground beef or ground turkey. Prep the beef or turkey, draining any excessive fat and set it aside. Select the Green Giant Steamer Vegetables and microwave and put in a bowl. Put a small bowl of cheese aside. Read the package for proper single serving for the cheese and use that amount in the potpie.

For easy prep, I mix the ingredients together in one bowl for the chicken potpie and one bowl for the Shepherd's potpie and set them aside. Take out the Pillsbury Crescent Rolls and potpie containers. I'd recommend spraying the containers with Pam for easy cleaning later.

Layer 7 cups with the pointed end of the triangular Crescent Roll and let the longer end hang over the edge. Fill each cup with the filling mix and spread the larger section of dough over the top. Pinch the sides so it stays in place and forms a crust over the top of the potpie.

If you have room in your freezer, make 14 cups, 7 chicken potpies and 7 Shepherd's potpies. If not, then do half and half of your choosing.

If you buy ready-cooked items, like the Green Giant Steamer Vegetables and the rotisserie chicken, the prep time is minimal. All you have to do is: cut up the chicken, cook the ground beef or ground turkey, heat the veggies, toss in a bowl with the soup mix and cheese (or layer cheese on top the potpie), layer container with the dough and bake.

Bake Time Warning: Crescent Rolls take longer to bake in the middle when they're on top a pie. I usually add 5-7 minutes to the package's recommended bake time. Make sure the crust is golden brown and, if necessary, use a fork to test.

SUBSTITUTE CRESCENT ROLLS
WITH BETTY CROCKER BISCUIT MIX

Calorie Count: See Chapters on Calorie Counts for Chicken Potpies and Shepherd's Pie. If you find your selection are totally over your daily caloric intake count for breakfast, lunch and dinner, then modify the recipes or use mini-containers (also available from Pantry Elements at Amazon.com).

Let baked items cool. You now have an entire, pre-packaged meal plan for a week and it only took around an hour. Note: It'll probably take longer the first time you do this because you'll need to get used to putting everything together, but once you get the hang of it; you'll be in and out of the kitchen with time to spare in the upcoming week because you won't have to cook!

After the items cool, cover and freeze. Each day remove, heat and eat. It's that simple. If you like the smell of potpies baking, you can freeze the pies unbaked and bake later, but this adds cooking time to your weekly schedule. Use only as an alternative on winter evenings to heat up your home and add the comforting smell of fresh, baked goods to the house.

If you grow tired of the crescent roll and biscuit crusts, get creative with alternate crust options (mentioned above), like:

CORNFLAKE CRUST
CRUSHED NUTS CRUST
FRUIT CRUST
LOW-FAT CHEESE CRUST

As long as you stick with lower fat options and keep the portion size down, then you can get creative with crusts. For higher calorie options, only add a crust to the top of the potpie.

SNACK ATTACK

Eating just potpies three times a day can become tedious. First, you're going to get hungry between meals. I think the simplest approach to snacks is to stick with fruits and dairy. I have an apple for my morning snack and a ¼ cup low-fat cottage cheese for my afternoon snack. You can mix and match fruits and dairy. There are plenty of low-fat milk options, yogurts, but watch the calorie count.

I also advocate adding a mixed green salad to the lunch and dinner potpie meals. Keep it simple and only use low-calorie, low-fat dressings. Restrict the salad to veggies and don't add extras, like cheese, eggs or meats.

WHAT ABOUT DESSERT?

I don't want to burn you out on making potpies, but if you really want to push the comfort limits, then make mini-fruit cobblers using canned pie fillings and the crescent rolls or biscuit mix. It's recommended that you substitute half the canned pie filling with fresh fruit to offset the fat and calorie count. Bake, cool, freeze and enjoy. The key to eating this type of dessert without breaking the diet bank is the word 'mini' – make the cobblers in cupcake tins to make sure the portion size is just right. Do NOT use the potpie containers.

If the fruit cobblers break the diet bank or you don't want to take the extra time to make them, then stick with traditional options, like diet Jell-O with a dollop of whipped crème topping (25 calories) or eat a piece of fruit or if you find you're really hungry in the evening, try a celery stick with a teaspoon of peanut butter. The protein in the peanut butter should satisfy the hunger. However, I think you'll find the comforting foods provided in The Potpie will fill you up, keep you from having cravings and keep the hunger pangs at bay.

LOW-CARB ALTERNATIVES

If you're still stuck on believing you can only lose weight by cutting carbs and you're concerned about the dough in the potpies, then use other crust options:

LOW-FAT CHEESE
EGG WHITES
GROUND /TURKEY TOPPING
GROUND OR CHOPPED NUTS

Do the prep as outlined in this book, but substitute the Pillsbury, refrigerated dough for the Low-Carb Alternatives listed above or come up with creative alternatives of your own. Be sure to watch the calorie count because low-carb doesn't always mean low fat or low-calorie.

QUANTITY FACTOR

The prep offered in the book covers 7 days (1 week), but you can easily expand it to 2 weeks or even a month. For the long, wintry months, my great grandmother often prepped and froze meals a month ahead. This will require more prep time and a lot more freezer room, but in the long run you can save a tremendous amount of time and money.

CHAPTER 5

EATING OUT

FAST FOOD CRUNCH

There's nothing quite like the experience of a drive-thru. Talk about convenient. You don't even have to get out of your car. In fact, you can eat in the car! Fast food is an American past time because it fits our busy lifestyles by saving us time, but usually at the expense of healthy eating. However, some fast food establishments have made an effort to put healthier choices on the menu. But let's face it; if you're in the drive-thru line, you're probably not there for the apple and walnut salad. Your mind's set on a juicy burger with an extra large French fry and a Coca-Cola.

What are doing there in the first place? Aren't you supposed to be dieting? If you find yourself visiting the fast food lane and you aren't there because your boss had a craving for a Big Mac, then you've probably grown tired of the diet plan. You start to justify how dieting is stupid because the very word has 'die' in it and you're tired of being hungry. So you binge and eat enough calories for three days. I won't even haggle you over the fat content. We'll just say it's way too much and leave it at that.

Hitting the fast food lane doesn't have to be the end of your diet. Consider it a temporary sidetrack that won't hurt once in a while. To be deprived of fast food forever is ridiculous. Besides, most of us want what we can't have. And if you believe you can't have fast food, then that's what you'll want!

But at least try to make a healthier selection. Instead of the double cheeseburger or even the cheeseburger, pick the hamburger with ketchup instead of mayo. Skip the fries and select a juice or diet soda for the beverage.

My favorite thing is McDonald's breakfast, but instead of the Egg McMuffin with the crazy-high calories and fat, I order a side of scrambled eggs and a side of bacon. This is lower calories, lower fat and for those watching carbs, it's the ideal choice. Guess what? You just ate out without breaking your diet! I'd also like to mention that burger joints like In-N-Out (West Coast USA) and Carl's Jr. offer a low-carb burger wrapped in lettuce instead of the bun. At Carl's, go for the grilled chicken burger instead of the beef and save on calories.

This isn't an excuse to eat out everyday, but it'll help on those days when your taste buds need a change or you need a change. And you won't have to feel guilty afterwards.

Besides, the objective of the Potpie Diet is help you save time and money while you lose weight. Eating out every day can sabotage time, money and weight loss efforts.

RESTAURANT VISITS

I bet you love to go out to a nice, sit-down dinner. Doesn't everyone? The great thing about restaurant visits is that you'll most likely know where you're going ahead of time, so you can pre-plan. Look up the restaurant on-line. Most restaurants list their menu and a nutritional guide on their website. Decide what you're going to have before arriving at the restaurant.

I recommend going with the 500 calories or under selections often found in the 'Lighter Choices' part of the menu. Most restaurants have these options available in a variety of foods from salads to chicken, fish and beef selections. The key is to plan ahead.

Dessert disaster! Oh no, you've already eaten your total daily calorie allowance and your gal pal wants to split a dessert. Go for it! But ask if the gal pal will split a shooter-size dessert or a dessert with slightly less guilt associated with it. Personally, I hate when I go out with friends who know I'm dieting and want to tempt me or sabotage my efforts by coaxing me in to splitting a dessert or having dessert at all. I usually just turn them down, but I know it's very hard. Like the meal, try to plan dessert ahead. Maybe leave 100-200 calories for a dessert, order a 500-calories dessert and only eat 1/3 of it. I know it's wasteful, but it's better left on the plate than on your hips.

*HAVE YOUR DESSERT
AND DIET TOO*

And your friends will never be able to sabotage your efforts again because you've outsmarted them.

STALLONE FACTOR

Some years ago I was reading how Sylvester Stallone stays in shape. Besides the obvious body building workouts he undergoes on a regular basis, he takes off one day a week and eats whatever he wants. I don't think there's anything wrong with taking a day off, but don't make it an excuse to binge.

Think of it as a Wild Card Diet Day. Maybe you'll have a standard McDonald's diet breakfast with a side of scrambled eggs and bacon, then you'll have a low-carb burger for lunch, then a sensible dinner.

The key to the Wild Card Day is to eat at least one sensible meal during this day or make alternate choices, like the low-carb burger instead of the regular burger.

CHAPTER 6

QUITTING THE DIET

NO MORE POTPIES

You've been doing The Potpie Diet for three months, you've lost weight and you're looking and feeling great, but you have to admit that you've had it with potpies!

First, The Potpie Diet isn't meant to make you eat potpies your entire life. It's meant to help you save time, money and learn to properly portion meals so you can lose weight. The time and money factors come into play because you're pre-making foods to eat for a week and saving money by eating your own foods instead of going out or eating pre-packaged foods that may not be good for you.

Mix things up! First, don't go cold turkey. Instead of 2 potpies a day, reduce to 1 for the first week or two. For example, replace your lunch chicken potpie with a chicken breast salad with light dressing. A week later, you can do the same for dinner. You can always go back to the pre-made, time and money saving potpies whenever you like.

If I find myself getting bored with the potpies, I keep my fast, on-the-go breakfast selection egg wraps and eat a sensible lunch and dinner with reasonable snacks. Then in a few weeks, I go back to the potpies for a few months. Mix and match options, always remembering to stay within the daily caloric intake and eat in proportionally smaller amounts with healthier choices.

You can always go back to the convenience of The Potpie Diet anytime you want to.

POTPIE PARTY

Or better than quitting cold turkey, gather your friends and have a potpie party! They keep asking how you lost weight. Show them! Instead of a salad bar or ice cream bar, you'll have a potpie bar! Your guests can select their favorite foods, make their own pies and bake them in the oven. It's a fun way to spend an afternoon and you'll get new ideas. Did Carol just mix cranberries in her chicken potpie? Did Dan add asparagus to his egg and turkey sausage wraps?

The new ideas will inspire you to keep going while sharing the gift of fast and convenient weight loss with friends. Everyone tells friends how they lost weight, but now you can show them!

CHAPTER 7

SAMPLE MEAL PLANS

(NOTE: DAILY CALORIE COUNTS DO NOT INCLUDE BEVERAGES)

MONDAY – CRUNCH DAY

It's time to get back to your weekly routine with the kids, work, driving, meetings and errands. There's no time to waste. You already prepped your potpie meals, so here's a sample menu to get you started. Modify according to your daily caloric intake.

	CALORIES
BREAKFAST 1 Egg, Turkey Sausage & Cheese Wrap (See Chapter 8 for Recipe)	130
SNACK 1 Small Apple ¼ Cup Low-Fat, Small Curd Cottage Cheese	55 130
LUNCH Mini Roasted Vegetable Potpie (See Chapter 8 for Recipe) Tossed Green Salad w/ Balsamic Vinaigrette	210 60
SNACK ½ Cup Low-Fat Milk Berry Flavored Fruit Roll up – 1 Qty.	65 104
DINNER Chicken Potpie (See Chapter 8 for Recipe)	330
DESSERT ½ Celery Stick w/ 1 tsp. Peanut Butter	97
TOTAL	**1181 Calories**

TUESDAY – SPAGHETTI DAY

You've starting to get the hang of how easy, fast and fun The Potpie Diet is. You love the comfort foods. You love the time and money saved. Keep it going! Here's another sample menu. Modify according to your daily caloric intake.

	CALORIES
BREAKFAST 1 Small Apple ¼ Cup Low-Fat, Small Curd Cottage Cheese	55 130
SNACK 1 Egg, Turkey Sausage & Cheese Wrap (See Chapter 8 for Recipe)	130
LUNCH Betty Crocker Biscuit Vegetable Potpie (See Chapter 8 for Recipe)	200
SNACK ½ Cup Low-Fat Milk ½ Cup Red or Green Grapes	65 55
DINNER Spaghetti & Meatball Potpie (See Chapter 8 for Recipe) Tossed Green Salad w/ Balsamic Vinaigrette	410 60
DESSERT Sugar Free Jell-O Cup w/ a Dollop of Reddi Whip	25
TOTAL	**1130 Calories**

WEDNESDAY – HAMBURGER & FRIES DAY

It's the middle of the week and you're doing great. Best of all, you're not feeling hungry! You've learned how to modify comfort foods so you can eat them every single day! Modify according to your daily caloric intake.

	CALORIES
BREAKFAST 1 Egg, Turkey Sausage & Cheese Wrap (See Chapter 8 for Recipe)	130
SNACK Low-fat, Light Yoplait Yogurt Cup ½ Celery Stick w/ tsp. Peanut Butter	110 97
LUNCH Hamburger & Fries Potpie (See Chapter 8 for Recipe)	340
SNACK ½ Cup Low-Fat Milk ½ Orange	65 55
DINNER Crescent Roll Turkey Potpie (See Chapter 8 for Recipe)	220
DESSERT Sugar Free Jell-O Cup w/ a Dollop of Reddi Whip	25
TOTAL	**1042 Calories**

THURSDAY – PEACH COBBLER DAY

We all love peach cobbler! It's been a long, hard week and you deserve a treat. Enjoy. Here's another sample menu. Modify according to your daily caloric intake.

	CALORIES
BREAKFAST 1 Small Apple Low-Fat, Light Yoplait Yogurt Cup	55 110
SNACK 1 Egg, Turkey Sausage & Cheese Wrap (See Chapter 8 for Recipe)	130
LUNCH Betty Crocker Biscuit Vegetable Potpie (See Chapter 8 for Recipe)	200
SNACK ½ Celery Stick w/ 1 tsp Peanut Butter	97
DINNER Betty Crocker Biscuit Chicken Potpie (See Chapter 8 for Recipe)	220
DESSERT Mini Peach Cobbler w/ Dollop of Reddi Whip (See Chapter 8 for Recipe)	210
TOTAL	**1022 Calories**

FRIDAY – PIZZA FOR BREAKFAST

You need something out of the norm to keep you from feeling like you're dieting. It's time to go crazy and have pizza for breakfast. Eat it cold or eat it hot! Here's another sample menu. Modify according to your daily caloric intake.

	CALORIES
BREAKFAST 1 Crescent Roll Slice Pizza (See Chapter 8 for Recipe)	320
SNACK Sugar Free Jell-O Cup w/ a Dollop of Reddi Whip 1 Small Peach	25 31
LUNCH Betty Crocker Biscuit Tuna Potpie (See Chapter 8 for Recipe)	280
SNACK ¼ Cup Low-Fat, Small Curd Cottage Cheese ½ Large Apple	130 55
DINNER Crescent Roll Chicken Potpie (See Chapter 8 for Recipe) Tossed Green Salad w/ Balsamic Vinaigrette	210 60
DESSERT ½ Cup Low-Fat Chocolate Milk	130
TOTAL	**1241 Calories**

SATURDAY – WILD CARD DAY

It's time to take most of the day off from potpies. You're even going to eat out! Here's a sample menu for eating out. Modify according to your daily caloric intake and be sure to read Chapter 5: Eating Out.

	CALORIES
BREAKFAST @ McDonalds McDonald's Side Order – Scrambled Eggs McDonald's Side Order - Sausage	 160 174
SNACK 1 Small Apple	 55
LUNCH Carl's Jr 1/3 lb. Low-Carb Hamburger (With no Mayo or Cheese)	 360
SNACK ½ Orange	 50
DINNER Betty Crocker Biscuit Chicken Potpie (See Chapter 8 for Recipe) Tossed Green Salad w/ Balsamic Vinaigrette	 220 60
DESSERT Sugar Free Jell-O Cup w/ a Dollop of Reddi Whip	 25
TOTAL	**1104 Calories**

SUNDAY – SHEPHERD'S POTPIE DAY

It's a day to rest and relax, so get back to The Potpie Diet to save time. Enjoy the day! Here is another sample menu. Modify according to daily caloric intake.

	CALORIES
BREAKFAST 1 Egg, Turkey Sausage & Cheese Wrap (See Chapter 8 for Recipe)	130
SNACK ½ Celery Stick w/ 1 tsp. Peanut Butter ½ Cup Low-Fat Milk	97 65
LUNCH Betty Crocker Biscuit Chicken Potpie (See Chapter 8 for Recipe) Tossed Green Salad w/ Balsamic Vinaigrette	220 60
SNACK Low-Fat, Light Yoplait Yogurt Cup	110
DINNER Shepherd's Potpie (See Chapter 8 for Recipe)	460
DESSERT ½ Cup Low-Fat Chocolate Milk	95
TOTAL	**1237 Calories**

CHAPTER 8

RECIPES

EGG, TURKEY SAUSAGE & CHEESE WRAP
(Modify recipe by using lean
bacon instead of turkey sausage)

1-Package, 8 Pillsbury Crescent Rolls
Egg whites from 7 eggs
Low-Fat, Sliced American Cheese
Jenny-O, Turkey Sausage Links (7 Total)

Cook turkey links, set aside. Cook egg whites, set aside. Separate Crescent rolls into 7, triangular sections (there will be one roll extra). Add sliced American Cheese Slices to each Crescent triangular roll, and then add egg whites and turkey sausage (dividing between the 7 rolls).

Heat oven to 400
Bake 15-18 minutes or until golden brown.
Cool on rack.
Wrap in freezer bags and freeze.
Heat in microwave 30 seconds – 1 minute, serve.

Calories per serving: 130
Serving Size: 1 Crescent Wrap

Note: Great breakfast for on-the-go families. Perfect for teens.

CRESCENT ROLL SLICE PIZZA
(Modify recipe for optional toppings; bacon, fruits)

1 Can Pillsbury, refrigerated Classic Pizza Crust
1 Bag (11.8 oz.) Green Giant Seasoned Steamers
½ Cup Basil Pesto
1 Cup Coarsely Chopped Kale (or Spinach)
4 oz. Prosciutto, chopped
2 Cups Shredded, Low-Fat Mexican Cheese Blend (8 oz.)
3 Eggs, well beaten

STEP 1
Heat oven to 400 degrees. Spray 13x9 pan with Pam. Unroll dough.
Press dough in pan ½ inch up sides. Bake for 7 minutes.

STEP 2
Microwave the Green Giant Seasoned Steamers Vegetables

STEP 3
Spread on ingredients

STEP 4
Bake 12-17 minutes or until golden brown and eggs separate
Cool 5 minutes.

Calories per serving: 320
Serving Size: 1 Slice, Even Cut Pizza from pan (1/8 of pan)
Pan makes approximately 10 servings, Cool and freeze 7 portions.

Note: This makes a nice, flatbread that can be used to make mini-
chicken, turkey ground beef or other alternative meals.

HAMBURGER & FRIES POTPIE
(Modify recipe w/ ground turkey)

1 ½ lbs. Lean Ground Beef (or Ground Turkey)
1 Large Onion, Chopped (1 cup)
2 Tablespoons, All-Purpose Flour
1 Can, Diced Tomatoes, Undrained
1 Cup Shredded, Low-Fat Cheddar Cheese (4 oz.)
2 Cups Frozen Crispy French Fries Potatoes (from 20 oz. bag)

Heat over 450 degrees.
Cook beef, onions and drain grease. Put in 12-inch, non-stick pan. Sprinkle with flour. Stir in tomatoes. Heat to boil.

Put equal amounts into 7 potpie containers. Layer top with frozen French fries and sprinkle with cheese.

Bake, uncovered 20 minutes until potatoes are golden brown. Cool, wrap and freeze.

Calories per serving: 340
Serving Size: 1 Potpie container

Note: Use ground turkey for a lower fat and calorie count. For lower carb count, use cheese topping only and do not use French fries.

BETTY CROCKER BISCUIT CHICKEN POTPIE
(Use instead of Pillsbury Crescent Rolls)

1 Cup Cut-Up Chicken
1 Bag (12 oz.) Green Giant Steamers
1 Can (10 3/4oz.) Condensed 98% Fat Free Cream of Chicken Soup
(Or use Cream of Mushroom)
½ Cup Fat Free (skim) Milk
1 Cup Biscuit Mix
½ Cup Fat Free (skim) Milk
1 Egg

Heat oven 400 degrees.
In ungreased, 2-quart casserole dish, mix chicken, vegetables, soup and ½ cup milk. Microwave on high for 4 minutes, stir.

In a small bowl, stir Biscuit mix, ½ cup milk and the egg with fork until blended.

Spoon chicken, vegetable and soup mix equally into 7 potpie containers. Cover each with Biscuit mix.

Bake uncovered about 30 minutes or until golden brown. Cool, wrap and freeze.

Note: Substitute chicken with ground turkey or even Tofu.

BETTY CROCKER BISCUIT VEGETABLE POTPIE
(Use instead of Pillsbury Crescent Rolls)

1 Cup Chopped-Up, Cooked Vegetables
1 Bag (12 oz.) Green Giant Steamers (optional)
1 Can (10 ¾ oz.) Condensed 98% Fat Free Cream of Chicken Soup
(Or use Cream of Mushroom)
½ Cup Fat Free (skim) Milk
1 Cup Biscuit Mix
½ Cup Fat Free (skim) Milk
1 Egg

Heat oven 400 degrees.
In ungreased, 2-quart casserole dish, mix fresh vegetables, soup and ½ cup milk. Microwave on high for 4 minutes, stir.

In a small bowl, stir Biscuit mix, ½ cup milk and the egg with fork until blended.

Spoon vegetables and soup mix equally into 7 potpie containers. Cover each with Biscuit mix.

Bake uncovered about 30 minutes or until golden brown. Cool, wrap and freeze.

Note: Substitute vegetable for Tofu for added protein. For extra flavor, use fresh peppers (green, yellow or red), roast on a Pam-sprayed cookie sheet with a dash of olive oil. Chop into pieces and use in place of the cooked vegetables, approximately 1 cup.

SHEPHERD'S POTPIE

1 Box Pillsbury, refrigerated piecrust, softened as directed on box
1 ½ cups Green Giant Steamers Mixed Vegetables
1 Tablespoon Butter (substitute with I Can't Believe It's Not Butter)
½ Medium Yellow Onion, Chopped
½ lb. Lean (80%) Ground Beef (or use Ground Turkey)
1/3 Cup Beef Broth
¼ tsp. Salt
1/8 tsp. Pepper
1 Bag (24 oz.) Mashed Potatoes (3 cups)

Heat oven to 400 degrees. Unroll piecrust. Roll each crust to 12-inches in diameter, cut into rounds to fit potpie containers. Spray containers with Pam. Firmly press dough into bottoms and up sides. Bake 7-10 minutes or until lightly browned. Remove from oven.

Reduce oven temperature to 350 degrees.

Heat vegetables in the microwave. Cook meat w/ onions and drain fat. Add broth, salt & pepper. Cook 3-5 minutes. Stir in vegetables.

Fill mixture into potpie cups and top with mashed potatoes, approximately ¼ cup each.

Bake 350 degrees 25-30 minutes or until crust brown and potatoes lightly browned. Remove from oven. Cool. Wrap and freeze.

Makes 12 servings
460 Calories per serving

CRESCENT ROLL CHICKEN POTPIE

1 Bag (16oz) Frozen Mixed Vegetables (Green Giant Variety)
2 Cups Cooked Chicken
1 Can (10 ¾ oz.) Condensed, Reduced-Fat Cream Chicken Soup
1 Can (10 ¾ oz.) Condensed, Cream of Mushroom Soup
1 Can (8 Rolls) Pillsbury, Refrigerated Crescent Dinner Rolls.

STEP 1

In a large bowl, mix vegetables, chicken and soups. Open Crescent Rolls and divide into 8 triangles.

STEP 2

Spray 7 potpie containers and press 1 Crescent Dinner Roll into each, with thin, triangular side on bottom. Allow wider side to hang over the side. Pour equal amounts of chicken mixture into cups and cover with remaining dough. Pinch dough on sides.

STEP 3

Bake 350 degrees 25-30 minutes or until crescent rolls are golden brown. Cooking times vary. Recommend using a fork to check the crescent roll on top of the potpie. Remove from oven. Cool, wrap and freeze.

Makes 7 servings.
Calories per serving: 270

Note: Substitute chicken with lean beef, lean ground beef, turkey or ground turkey.

MEXICAN BOWL POTPIE

1 Can (8oz) Pillsbury Crescent Recipe Creations, Refrigerated Seamless Dough (Or Pillsbury Crescent, Refrigerated Rolls)
2 Tablespoons Butter (Substitute w/ I Can't Believe It's Not Butter)
¼ Cup Chopped Onion
1 Tablespoon All-Purpose Flour
¼ tsp. Salt
1/8 tsp. Pepper
1 Cup Chicken Broth
1 Pkg (6 oz.) Refrigerated Chicken Breast Strips, Southwest, chopped
1 Can (15oz.) Black Beans, Drained
3 Tablespoons Old El Paso Canned Chopped Chilies, Drained
1 Cup Green Giant Frozen Corn
½ Cup Low-Fat, Shredded Cheddar Jack Cheese (2oz)
½ Cup Old El Paseo Thick n Chunky Salsa (Any Variety)

STEP 1 Heat oven to 350 degrees. Spray 7 potpie containers with Pam.

STEP 2 Unroll rough and shape into potpie containers. Stretch to fit.

STEP 3 Bake 12-15 minutes until golden brown. Cool 15 minutes.

STEP 4 In saucepan, melt butter over medium heat. Add onions, cook 2 minutes, and stir until tender. Add flour, salt & pepper and stir until well blended. Gradually stir in broth. Cook & stir until bubbly and thickened. Stir in chicken, black beans, green chilies and corn. Simmer 5 minutes or until hot.

STEP 5 Spoon equal amounts into potpie containers. Top with cheese and salsa. Pop in oven just long enough to melt cheese and make a cheesy crust. Remove from oven. Cool, wrap and freeze.

Makes 7 servings
Calories: 550 per serving

Note: Substitute chicken with ground turkey. Add taco-seasoning package to meat for an extra Mexican-style flavoring.

CRESCENT ROLL TURKEY POTPIE

1 ½ Cups Frozen Peas and Carrots
1 Cup Cubed (1/2 inch) Cooked Turkey
1 Cup Refrigerated cooked diced potatoes with onion (from 20oz frozen bag)
¼ Cup Low-Fat Milk
½ tsp. Dried Thyme Leaves
1 Can (10 ¾ oz.) Condensed Cream of Chicken Soup
1 Can (8 Rolls) Pillsbury, Refrigerated Crescent Dinner Rolls
1 Egg
1 Tablespoon Water
1/8 tsp. Dried Thyme Leaves

STEP 1
Heat oven 400 degrees. Mix peas & carrots, turkey, potatoes, milk, ½ teaspoon thyme and the soup. Heat to boiling over medium-high heat, stirring occasionally. Turn off and set aside.

STEP 2
Unroll dough into separate triangles. Spray potpie containers with Pam. Place 1 dough triangle with thin side down in the potpie container and leave wide part hanging over the edge. Fill equal amounts of turkey mixture into cups.

STEP 3
In a small bowl, mix egg and water. Cover potpie with remaining dough and pinch edges. Brush mixture over dough, sprinkle 1/8-teaspoon thyme over dough. Bake 11-13 minutes or until crusts are golden brown. Cooking times may vary up to 30 minutes because Crescent Rolls on top of the potpie often take longer to cook than on a cookie sheet. Use a fork to test the roll and leave in oven until it's golden brown. Cool, wrap and freeze.

Makes 7 Servings (Note: There will be one Crescent Roll left)
Calories per serving: 330

Note: Substitute Cream of Chicken Soup for Cream of Mushroom or Cream of Celery soups.

BETTY CROCKER BISCUIT TUNA POTPIE

1 Large Can Chunk White Tuna (in water)
1 Bag (12 oz.) Green Giant Steamers
1 Can (10 ¾ oz.) Condensed 98% Fat Free Cream of Chicken Soup
(Or use Cream of Mushroom)
½ Cup Fat Free (skim) Milk
1 Cup Biscuit Mix
½ Cup Fat Free (skim) Milk
1 Egg

Heat oven 400 degrees.
In ungreased, 2-quart casserole dish, mix tuna, vegetables, soup and ½ cup milk. Microwave on high for 4 minutes, stir.

In a small bowl, stir Biscuit mix, ½ cup milk and the egg with fork until blended.

Divide tuna, vegetable and soup mix into 7 potpie containers. Cover with Biscuit mix.

Bake uncovered about 30 minutes or until golden brown. Remove from oven. Cool, wrap and freeze.

Makes 7 Servings
Calories: 280 per serving

Note: Substitute tuna with ground turkey or even Tofu.

SPAGHETTI & MEATBALL POTPIE

1 Bag Pre-Cooked Turkey Meatballs
1 Medium-Large Spaghetti Squash
1 Jar Spaghetti Sauce (Original or Mushroom Flavor)
1 lb. Ground Turkey
1 Pkg. Spaghetti Sauce Mix
1 Small Onion
½ Pkg. Fresh, Sliced Mushrooms
1 Can (8 Rolls) Pillsbury, Refrigerated Crescent Dinner Rolls.

STEP 1
Heat oven to 400 degrees. Spray 7 potpie containers with Pam and set aside.

STEP 2
Steam spaghetti squash until tender. Use a fork and slice into long, thin spaghetti strands and set aside.

STEP 3
Cut up onion and mushroom. Cook with ground turkey until browned. Add in 1 Pkg. Spaghetti Sauce and mix into meat.

STEP 4
Heat spaghetti sauce and 7 turkey meatballs together in a saucepan.

STEP 5
Unroll Crescent Rolls. Place thin side down in containers and leave wide side hanging over the edge. Mix sauce, meat and spaghetti squash in a bowl. Add equal amounts of mixture in the 7-potpie containers. Cover with remaining dough and pinch dough to sides.

Bake 25-30 minutes until crescent rolls are golden brown. Cool, wrap and freeze.

Makes 7 servings.
Calories per serving: 410

MINI PEACH COBBLER

1 Can Peach Pie Filling
1 Cup Fat Free (skim) Milk
1 Cup Biscuit Mix
1 Egg

Heat oven 400 degrees. Use cupcake foils or paper cupcakes to make 7 mini cobblers. Arrange in a muffin pan.

In a small bowl, stir Biscuit mix, 1-cup milk and the egg with fork until blended. Pour just enough to cover bottom of muffin cup. Add equal amounts of Peach Pie Filling, and then cover with remaining Biscuit mix.

Bake 30 minutes or until golden brown. Cool, wrap and freeze.

Makes 7 Servings
Calories: 210 per serving

FINAL WORD

Dieting is hard, but why? Because you feel deprived of comfort foods. While you have to give up certain things, like junk food, The Potpie Diet allows you to eat the hearty meals you love.

This book has taught you how to modify the recipes for your favorite potpie meals, bake the proper portion-ready size, freeze and eat-on-demand to help you lose weight, maintain weight, save time and money! You finally have the lifestyle you deserve. You're on your way to a healthier you.

Best wishes always and enjoy your potpies!